Whitening Teeth

Quickly and Safely Whiten Your Teeth for a Permanently Brighter Smile!

BENJAMIN TIDEAS

CONTENTS

INTRODUCTION

I want to congratulate you for finding this book, "Whitening Teeth: Quickly and Safely Whiten Your Teeth for a Permanently Brighter Smile".

This book contains proven steps and strategies on how to make your teeth whiter, more vivid and improve your smile for life!

This will serve as a handy guide for those who wish to feel more confident about themselves by ensuring that they present a clean, white and beautiful set of teeth. This book contains a few pieces of advice designed to improve your oral and dental health and bring out your most radiant smile.

Thanks again for grabbing this book, I hope you enjoy it. Now, let's get to it!

FIRST IMPRESSIONS LAST

Some people view the process of undergoing teeth whitening procedures as being vain. However, one should realize that the procedure is extremely important in various aspects of your life. Having a bright and white set of teeth can help in improving your look. Keep in mind that first impressions last and you need to bring out a beautiful smile to create a lasting impression. Yellowed and stained teeth can prevent people from leaving a good impression especially when applying for a job, meeting new friends or impressing their dates. It can only make them feel self-conscious.

Fortunately, there are now a few solutions for yellowed and stained teeth. All it takes is to visit your dentist to determine which among the whitening solutions will work in your favor. There are also products that can be used in the comfort of your own home. Making great improvements in your teeth and smile works in bringing out a more confident you, regardless of the whitening method used. This can create a positive impact in various aspects of your life.

Primary Reasons for Stained and Yellowed Teeth

Understanding the primary reasons for obtaining a stained and yellowed set of teeth is often necessary before visiting your dentist and undergoing any whitening treatment. This is essential in understanding the main cause of teeth discoloration and finding the best way to deal with it. The foods and drinks you regularly consume play a major impact on the color of your teeth. Among the foods and drinks that cause staining are colas, tea, coffee, certain fruits and vegetables like potatoes and apples and wines.

Another reason for stained or yellowed teeth is the use of tobacco.

Chewing or smoking has the tendency of ruining your smile, so make sure to avoid doing this habit excessively. It is also necessary to follow a good dental hygiene regimen. Remember that poor oral and dental hygiene such as inadequate flossing and brushing might cause plaque and other substances that produce stains like tobacco and coffee to be left inside your mouth. This might lead to excessive tooth discoloration.

It should also be noted that there are certain diseases that can negatively affect the color of your tooth. This holds true for sufferers of diseases that greatly affect the enamel or the hard surface of one's tooth and dentin, or the underlying material found beneath the enamel. Treatments for the health conditions might also stain your teeth. For instance, chemotherapy and neck and head radiation might also result to losing the natural whiteness of your teeth

The use of certain dental materials can also influence your tooth's color. Dentistry materials like amalgam restorations including those that contain silver sulfide have the tendency of casting a gray-black color into your tooth. An advancing age can also lose its natural color. It can even make your set of teeth become yellowish. Genetics also play a significant role in tooth discoloration. Note that there are people who naturally and genetically have thicker and brighter enamel than others.

Tooth discoloration can also be triggered by excessive fluoride coming from a few environmental sources like the ones naturally found in water. Excessive fluoride utilization due to the regular use of fluoride rinses, applications, supplements and toothpaste can also trigger the staining. Trauma affecting the tooth such as the one caused by damages brought on by a fall might also disturb the formation of enamel especially in children, who are still on the stage of developing their teeth. This leads to discoloration.

It is crucial to gain an understanding about the different causes of tooth discoloration, staining and yellowing in both children and adults. It will be easy for anyone with stained teeth to find the right solutions in permanently restoring the beauty of ones teeth and smile by understanding the main causes of discoloration. This will be a good way to boost a person's confidence.

UNDERSTANDING THE DIFFERENT TYPES OF TOOTH DISCOLORATION

Your teeth have the tendency of becoming discolored over time because of numerous factors, like the ones mentioned in the first chapter. The discoloration might also start to develop in your jaws. It should be noted that there are various types of discoloration affecting one's teeth. It is vital to comprehend what form of discoloration affects your case since this works in finding the most suitable treatment.

Extrinsic / Outer Discoloration

This refers to stains found on the visible and outer surface of your teeth. It does not affect the actual underlying tooth color. The discoloration or acquired pellicle can be removed easily by polishing.

Here are few of the primary factors that cause extrinsic or outer discoloration:

- Coffee, particularly black coffee
- Black tea
- Red wine
- Some fruit juices like grapes and cranberry
- Dark cola beverages
- Certain foods like dark berries and curries
- Excessive smoking and chewing of tobacco
- Poor oral hygiene
- Iron supplements
- Chlorhexidine mouthwash

Intrinsic / Inner Discoloration

In this type, the actual substance of your tooth, primarily your dentin, alters its outer color. There are plenty of causes for this. One is your age. Your teeth tend to discolor naturally as you age. It is because the aging process might also cause your dentin to thicken and your enamel to become thin. Another factor that causes intrinsic discoloration is tetracycline, which is an antibiotic. Taking this antibiotic during the stage of forming dentition might cause them to look characteristically dark.

Nerve damage also has the tendency of triggering intrinsic discoloration. If the nerves found inside your teeth die due to decay or trauma, then the darkening of the affected teeth will follow. Nerve damage is one of the primary reasons why one or few of your teeth become discolored.

Intrinsic tooth discoloration is categorized in two groups. The first one is systemic, triggered either by defects or drugs. Note that the development of your dentition can be greatly affected by several systemic factors and metabolic conditions. The second one is the local group. An example of discoloration under this group is the one caused by root resorption, aging and pulpal hemorrhagic products.

Age Related Discoloration

This form of tooth discoloration is triggered by a combination of both intrinsic and extrinsic factors. Dentin tends to become naturally yellow over time. Your enamel, which works by covering your teeth, becomes thin as you age. Chips in your teeth or other dental injury can also cause their discoloration, especially if this damages your pulp.

A Few Prevention Tips

While stained and discolored teeth are common dental issues, be aware that there are a few ways to prevent it. One tip in preventing the buildup of stains is to reduce your intake or use of all the things that cause it, including the factors, foods, drinks and medications mentioned earlier in this book. Brushing two times a day can also help. However, dental experts do not recommend brushing teeth immediately after eating a meal. It is because this habit has the tendency of weakening your teeth structure over time. Instead of brushing, consider rinsing your mouth using water or a mouthwash after eating a big meal.

Seeking the aid of whitening toothpastes is also beneficial. Note that whitening toothpastes comprise of abrasives that work in boosting their ability to get rid of stains. However, despite the effectiveness of some whitening toothpastes in eradicating stains, these products are still incapable making changes into your interior tooth's shade. Changing your toothbrush after three months and using inter-dental brushes or floss to clean in between your teeth is also beneficial.

Allowing dental professionals to clean your teeth is also crucial in removing most of the staining that affect your smile and cause you to feel self-conscious. Seeking the help of dental professionals is often essential for those who deal with intrinsic discoloration since this means that the damage on your teeth has already been done. Since prevention is already too late for this case, the expert hands and knowledge of dental professionals are useful.

HOW TO WHITEN TEETH THE NATURAL WAY?

For those whose teeth have become stained or get discolored due to a number of uncontrollable factors, natural teeth whitening solutions will surely be the first treatments that will be sought. It is because these natural solutions are inexpensive, sometimes available right at home or in your kitchen, and are safe for almost all people. There are also natural teeth whitening solutions that work in permanently bringing out a naturally white set of teeth. All it takes is to choose one out of the many natural wonders that will perfectly work for your unique dental problem, and that you can tolerate.

Baking Soda

Baking soda is one of the most popular natural solutions for teeth whitening because of its ability to work as an antibacterial cleanser. It works in getting rid of tough stains found in a person's tooth by breaking them down. Using this natural product allows its molecules to establish a chemical reaction when these come into contact with the molecules present in the stain. Baking soda molecules attack stains in your teeth and break them apart. It also has abrasive particles that work in polishing the surface aside from lightening the stains.

The good thing about baking soda is that it is easy to use when it comes to whitening your teeth. Dipping your toothbrush into it and using it as your toothpaste can help. There are also toothpastes in the market that contain baking soda. Switching to this toothpaste can lighten the shade of your teeth.

Foods Rich in Cellulose

Foods such as apples, celery, and carrots are useful for those who deal with tooth discoloration because their high cellulose content increase their capability to work as safe and natural abrasives that cleanse your teeth and naturally remove surface stains. Greens including broccoli, lettuce, and spinach are also rich in mineral compounds that have the ability of forming a film over your affected teeth. This prevents the pigments coming from the other foods you eat from staining. Crunchy foods and veggies like cucumbers, celery and carrots also work in removing chemicals and sugars causing the cavities and stains.

Fruits with Tooth Whitening Capacity

There are a few fruits that are capable of naturally whitening your teeth, and eating them on a regular basis can help in maintaining a beautiful smile. These fruits work as excellent bleaches or whiteners. An example of this is strawberry which contains whitening agents. To take advantage of the teeth whitening ability of strawberry, you just have to rub it into your teeth. Creating toothpaste out of strawberry is also possible.

Strawberries also work as powerful teeth whiteners because these are rich in Vitamin C and astringent. Vitamin C aids in teeth whitening because it clears plaque away while the presence of astringent helps in eliminating surface stains. Just make sure to brush your teeth right after rubbing the fruit because this is also rich in sugar and acid that might harm them, in the long run.

Eating raisins can also help because it stimulates the production of saliva. This allows your teeth to be constantly washed, thereby rinsing the plaque and preventing the buildup.

Eating a crunchy apple is beneficial in naturally treating discolored teeth because it works similarly to a toothbrush upon chewing on it. This fruit helps in removing excess bacteria and food found in your mouth. It is also efficient in scrubbing away surface stains. It has Malic acid, which is a vital chemical used in various teeth whitening products. This acid is also useful in dissolving stains.

Regular Flossing and Brushing

This helps in preventing tooth discoloration, and regular flossing and brushing work in whitening and cleaning your teeth. Failing to perform this habit regularly might result in tooth decay and staining, which will further lead to discoloration. Both are also helpful in removing stains found in between your teeth. Aside from maintaining a bright smile, both flossing and brushing are also beneficial in improving the health of your gums and preventing diseases that affect them.

EFFECTIVE TEETH WHITENING PRODUCTS

Various teeth whitening products are now available in the market including over-the-counter gels, toothpastes, trays, rinses, strips and other whitening products offered by a dentist. It is for you to choose which one is right for your needs. The products are perfect for those who have unrestored teeth or those without fillings and who have healthy gums. People whose teeth are already yellowing and staining respond to these products the best.

Whitening Toothpastes

All toothpastes have the ability of removing surface stains due to their mild abrasives content. Some toothpastes, designed to whiten and brighten a person's teeth, have gentle chemical or polishing agents that further improve the effectiveness of the products in getting rid of stains. Most of these toothpastes also contain hydrogen peroxide that works efficiently in lightening the dark or yellow color visible in your tooth. These have the capacity of lightening the color of your teeth by a single shade.

Whitening toothpastes also utilize special abrasives that are effective in boosting its ability to get rid of surface stains. The special abrasives used are also finer versions of the ones utilized in standard toothpastes, so one can expect these to help in minimizing the risk of dealing with excessive tooth wear. However, one should realize that its effectiveness only works for surface stains, so dental professionals do not still recommend using the whitening toothpaste as a substitute for getting regular professional dental cleanings.

Whitening Gels and Strips

Whitening gels used to lighten the shade of your teeth refer to peroxide-based and clear gels applied directly into surfaces with the help of a small brush. Instructions for these over-the-counter gels often require direct application for two times daily, within fourteen days. The good thing about using the gels is that these are capable of showing results within just several days of use. Its results are also sustainable for up to four months.

Whitening strips refer to virtually invisible and thin strips coated with the help of a whitening gel based on peroxide. Using the products require application for two times daily for approximately thirty minutes. An advantage of these strips is that these are inexpensive and easy to use. It should be noted that the results will be visible within a few weeks. The results will also be dependent upon the level of strength of its peroxide.

Whitening Rinses

Whitening rinses form part of the newly introduced teeth whitening products in the market. These work similarly to mouthwashes, since they are capable of freshening your breath while also reducing your risk of dealing with gum diseases and dental plaque. However, many users view the rinses as more beneficial than mouthwashes because aside from performing the functions of the latter, the rinses also contain hydrogen peroxide that act as a teeth whitener.

In most cases, it will take around twelve weeks to notice results after starting to use the rinses. One just needs to swish the rinse around his or her mouth two times a day, for approximately sixty seconds. It is necessary to use it before brushing your teeth.

Teeth Whitening Pen

A teeth whitening pen is one of the most efficient ways of whitening your teeth. One thing that makes the product beneficial is the convenience involved when it comes to using it. The active ingredient of the pen is similar to the one used by other teeth whitening products, which boosts its ability to work. You just have to make sure to let the pen coat each tooth evenly and keep it in contact with your teeth.

Tray Based Whitening

The properly fitting mouth tray is an example of this. A tray based whitening product refers to a customized night guard which holds a gel. You need to wear it for a specified period, preferably around ten to fourteen days. The required period to wear this product will be dependent upon the peroxide gel concentration and type. Make sure to choose one which perfectly fits your mouth, to avoid problems when using it.

IN-OFFICE TEETH WHITENING

This option refers to professional teeth whitening procedures and methods done in a dental office. This is one of the most preferred whitening solutions of those who have yellowish and staining teeth. Aside from being performed by an expert dental professional, it also involves the application of strong agents into your affected tooth and gums. The most efficient whitening systems used in a dental clinic feature a buffer found in the gel. This offers utmost protection for your tooth enamel, so expect the procedure to be completed without causing damage to your oral and dental health.

The good thing about in-office teeth whitening is that it can make great improvements within just one office visit. Expect your teeth to brighten or lighten by up to ten shades within just one hour. In-office whitening covers only the eight teeth found in front. Undergoing the procedure is a good way to jump-start your decision to try at-home teeth whitening. This has an impact in making a whitening program effective.

Your dentist is the most qualified professional who can handle issues arising from the use of whitening treatments like tooth sensitivity. The whitening procedure conducted by a dental professional is capable of lasting for at least one year. This will be dependent upon the manner through which you take good care of your teeth. Its results will also last long if the health of your teeth is regularly maintained, and you combine it with the use of the most suitable at-home whitening product for your case.

In-Office Bleaching

This is one of the many dental procedures done in the clinic of your dentist. It works in restoring the brightness or lightness of your teeth. Procedures related to in-office bleaching involve the use of a protective layer cured by light. It also involves painting the protective layer into your papilla or the tips of your gums found between your teeth and your gums. This is beneficial in minimizing the risk of causing chemical burns into your soft tissues.

It uses a bleaching agent which is either hydrogen peroxide or carbamide peroxide that works by breaking down into your mouth in order to produce hydrogen peroxide. There are also in-office bleaching procedures that involve placing a protective gel or rubber guard into your gums in order to offer protection against irritation. Your dentist will then apply a peroxide gel into a tray which is custom-molded. This tray will be placed into your affected teeth.

Internal Bleaching

Internal bleaching is crucial for devitalized teeth that took endodontic treatment, but still obtained stains and discoloration because of the internal staining found in your tooth structure through blood and any other leaked fluids. What makes internal bleaching beneficial is that it works in brightening your teeth including its interiors.

Internally bleaching your teeth also involves drilling a hole into the pulp chamber, sealing, cleaning it up and filling your root canal using a substance which is quite similar to rubber. It also directly places a peroxide gel into the pulp chamber. This makes it possible for the procedure to work directly in the interiors of your tooth, specifically the dentin layer. It works in lightening teeth inside and out, so expect to obtain a bright smile after undergoing the procedure.

Laser Whitening

Laser whitening refers to one of the fastest procedures of all the teeth whitening solutions offered to the public. It normally takes around ninety minutes and uses a simple procedure. The laser teeth whitening session starts by covering and protecting your gums and lips with the help of a rubber shield. This can help in exposing only your teeth. Your dentist will then apply the bleaching agent or gel into your exposed teeth and use a specially designed light to boost the effectiveness of the product.

The use of both the laser light and bleaching gel works in penetrating into your teeth. The combination breaks up discoloration and stain. The laser light is highly efficient when it comes to activating the chemical found in the gel. Expect the procedure to work faster than bleaching alone.

BLEACHING PRODUCTS

Bleaching products refer to peroxide-based products that have the ability of altering the color of your teeth. Keep in mind, however, that not all forms of tooth discoloration can positively respond to the use of bleaching products. People who intend to use tooth bleaching should visit their dentist and seek consultation to figure out the main cause of their problem, and identify the best bleaching solution which can produce the most desirable results. This step is especially necessary for individuals who have root canal treatments, excessively dark and stained anterior teeth, crowns and fillings.

Your dentist might also be able to perform a variety of bleaching techniques and use different bleaching products. One method is vital bleaching, which your chosen dental professional will perform on a living tooth. It is useful in whitening surfaces that receive stains due to tobacco and certain foods, and those that have darkened due to age. Non-vital bleaching is another method, and this is useful on non-living teeth. It has the ability of lightening the color of your teeth from the inside out, especially if their color has changed due to a root canal.

The results produced by the use of a bleaching method or product will depend upon a few factors. These include the number of teeth that require bleaching and the severity of the staining or discoloration. To guarantee positive results, consider getting the treatment under the care and supervision of a licensed dentist. Professional teeth bleaching performed inside a dental clinic is safe and effective. It is because dental professionals are already well-trained and highly skillful when it comes to performing the procedures, especially the ones executed with the help of lights and laser.

Other Valuable Teeth Whitening Products

New and highly advanced teeth whitening products continue to pop out in the market including the newest versions of mouthwashes, dental floss and whitening chewing gum containing substances and ingredients that work in making positive changes in the color of your tooth. It is best to study the effectiveness of all these products prior to using any of them. A wise tip is to visit your dentist and find out if he can recommend an inexpensive yet highly effective product which will work in your particular case.

If your dentist performs a procedure to lighten your teeth, then make sure to follow-up the treatment by regularly visiting his clinic and adhering to his instructions when it comes to caring for your teeth when you are at home. Some dentists will recommend placing a whitening product into the teeth of their patients while they are at home. Follow the instructions of your dentist in this case to boost your chances of receiving your desired results.

It should also be noted that while dental treatments ideal for whitening are sometimes expensive, they are beneficial because they can last for a long time. Some can be expected to last for up to three years while others can permanently brighten your teeth and smile.

How to Preserve the Brightness of your Teeth after the Treatment

Taking good care of your oral and dental health can go a long way, when it comes to ensuring that the results of your teeth whitening treatment become permanent. A wise tip is to combine the use of other at-home whitening products with some positive changes in your diet and lifestyle, after undergoing a dental whitening treatment. Minimizing your use of tobacco products and consumption of black tea, coffee, red wine, grape juice and other drinks that can cause staining is a must.

It is also crucial to brush your teeth after drinking a beverage that triggers discoloration. Maintain their whiteness by also using the recommended whitening mouthwash and toothpaste by your dentist. Make sure to receive professional dental cleanings semi-annually since this is valuable in extending the life of the whitening treatments used in your case.

Aside from preserving your tooth's brightness, professional dental cleanings also work in preventing dental problems such as gum diseases and infections. By doing all these things, saying goodbye to stained and discolored teeth is within your reach! This can bring out permanently white teeth that can help in boosting your confidence and enhancing your look.

CONCLUSION

I want to personally Thank You again for reading this book!

I sincerely hope the information contained will help you to achieve the smile you desire and deserve by getting those pearly whites even whiter! An improved smile with whiter teeth not only improves your image, but also improves your self-confidence.

The next step is to put into practice the methods and employ the strategies we've discussed here to begin taking that brighter smile to the next level. Get started now!

Finally, if you enjoyed this book, please take the time to share your thoughts and post a positive review on Amazon. I would greatly appreciate your support!

Thank you and good luck!

Benjamin Tideas

Check out my other books and receive notifications to get my books for FREE!
www.plaid-enterprises.com

www.ingramcontent.com/pod-product-compliance
Lightning Source LLC
Chambersburg PA
CBHW071352310526
45790CB00018B/1429